BREASTFEEDING

AND

WOMEN'S

HEALTH

By

OLUCHI ONYEMAECHI OKEH

TABLE OF CONTENTS

INTRODUCTION

Breastfeeding and Women's Health

Breastfeeding is a remarkable natural process that has been nurturing infants for centuries. It not only provides essential nourishment for the baby but also holds immense benefits for the mother's health. Understanding the significance of breastfeeding for both the baby and the mother is vital in promoting optimal well-being for both.

In this comprehensive book, titled "Breastfeeding and Women's Health," we delve into the profound impact of breastfeeding on women's health. We explore the intricate connection between breastfeeding and its influence on various aspects of mother's physical, emotional, and mental well-being. From the early postpartum period to long-term effects, we aim to shed light on the myriad ways in which breastfeeding contributes to the overall health of women.

The First section of this book focuses on the importance of breastfeeding for both the baby's and the mother's health. We delve into the unparalleled benefits of breast milk, which is uniquely tailored to meet the nutritional needs of infants. Breast milk not only provides essential nutrients but also offers antibodies and enzymes that strengthen the baby's immune system, protecting against a myriad of diseases. We explore how breastfeeding establishes a strong bond between the mother and her child, fostering emotional connection and promoting healthy brain development in infants.

Additionally, we highlight the various ways in which breastfeeding benefits the mother, including promoting postpartum healing, reducing the risk of certain cancers, and supporting weight loss.

Moving on to second section, our primary focus is to explore the impact of breastfeeding on women's health. We delve into the physiological changes that occur in a woman's body during breastfeeding, such as hormonal fluctuations and their effects on mood and mental well-being. We examine the potential long-term benefits of breastfeeding, such as reduced risk of osteoporosis and cardiovascular disease. Furthermore, we shed light on the potential challenges and concerns women may face during their breastfeeding journey, such as lactation difficulties and postpartum depression, providing strategies and resources to overcome them.

With this book, we aim to empower women with knowledge and understanding, enabling them to make informed decisions about breastfeeding and its impact on their health. Whether you are an expectant mother, a new mother navigating the early days of breastfeeding, or someone interested in women's health, this book serves as a valuable resource to navigate the multifaceted relationship between breastfeeding and overall well-being.

Join us in this insightful journey as we unravel the remarkable connection between breastfeeding and women's health. Discover the power of this natural act and embrace the benefits it holds for both you and your child.

CHAPTER 1

Benefits of Breastfeeding for Women's Health

During the introduction, we explored the many advantages of breastfeeding for infant health. However, breastfeeding doesn't only benefit babies; it also has numerous positive effects on women's health. In this chapter, we will be learning the various physical and emotional benefits of breastfeeding for mothers.

A. Physical Benefits:

Promotes Postpartum Recovery:

Breastfeeding plays a crucial role in the postpartum recovery process. During pregnancy, a woman's body undergoes significant changes to support the growing baby. After childbirth, breastfeeding stimulates the release of oxytocin, a hormone that helps the uterus contract and returns to its pre-pregnancy size. This contraction reduces postpartum bleeding and aids in a faster recovery.

Reduces the Risk of Certain Cancers:

Breastfeeding offers remarkable protective benefits against certain types of cancers, primarily breast and ovarian cancer. Women who breastfeed their babies have a lower risk of developing breast cancer later in life. The longer the duration of breastfeeding, the greater the risk reduction. Additionally, breastfeeding has been found to reduce the risk of ovarian cancer, making it a valuable preventive measure for women.

Helps with Weight Loss:

One of the positive side effects of breastfeeding is its ability to assist women in shedding those extra pounds gained during pregnancy. Breastfeeding burns calories as the body produces milk. This calorie expenditure can contribute to gradual weight loss, especially when combined with a balanced diet and moderate exercise. By engaging in breastfeeding, mothers have a natural means to aid in their post-pregnancy weight management.

B. Emotional Benefits:

Enhances Bonding Between Mother and Baby:

Breastfeeding provides a unique opportunity for mothers to bond with their infants on a deep emotional level. The skin-to-skin contact, eye contact, and physical closeness during breastfeeding release hormones like prolactin and oxytocin, which promote feelings of love, affection, and attachment. This nurturing experience creates a strong emotional connection between mother and baby, fostering a sense of security and trust.

Reduces the Risk of Postpartum Depression and Anxiety:

Postpartum depression and anxiety are common mental health challenges that affect many women after childbirth. However, breastfeeding has been shown to lower the risk of developing these conditions. The release of oxytocin during breastfeeding helps to reduce stress levels, regulate mood, and create a sense of calm. Moreover, the intimate bond established through breastfeeding can provide emotional support, alleviating feelings of isolation and sadness.

Boosts Self-Esteem and Confidence:

Breastfeeding can significantly boost a mother's self-esteem and confidence. The ability to provide nourishment and sustenance to their baby can instill a sense of accomplishment and empowerment. Overcoming challenges associated with breastfeeding, such as latching difficulties or milk supply concerns, can enhance a mother's belief in her capabilities and strengthen her self-confidence. This newfound confidence often extends beyond breastfeeding, positively influencing other areas of a woman's life.

Conclusion:

Breastfeeding offers an array of physical and emotional benefits for women's health. From aiding postpartum recovery to reducing the risk of certain cancers, breastfeeding provides tangible advantages that contribute to a woman's overall well-being. Additionally, the emotional benefits, including enhanced bonding, reduced risk of postpartum depression and anxiety, and increased self-esteem and confidence, further emphasize the importance of breastfeeding as a transformative experience for both mother and baby.

CHAPTER 2

Breastfeeding Challenges and Solutions

Introduction:

Breastfeeding is a natural and beneficial way to nourish and bond with your baby. However, it is not always a smooth journey. Many women encounter challenges along the way that can make breastfeeding a daunting task. In this chapter, we will explore some common breastfeeding challenges and provide you with practical solutions to overcome them. By understanding these challenges and implementing effective strategies, you can enhance your breastfeeding experience and promote your overall health and well-being.

A. Common Breastfeeding Challenges

Sore Nipples and Breasts:

One of the most common challenges faced by breastfeeding mothers is sore nipples and breasts. This can be caused by improper latching, inadequate positioning, or sensitivity to the baby's sucking. It is important to address this issue early on to prevent further discomfort and potential complications.

Solution:

i. Ensure proper latching: Make sure your baby's mouth is wide open, covering not only the nipple but also a significant portion of the areola. This will promote effective milk transfer and reduce nipple soreness.

ii. Use nipple creams and ointments: Applying lanolin or other nipple creams after each feeding can soothe and moisturize the nipples, promoting healing and preventing further soreness.

iii. Air dry and wear loose clothing: After each feeding, allow your nipples to air dry and wear loose, breathable clothing to minimize friction and irritation.

Low Milk Supply or Oversupply:

Another challenge faced by breastfeeding mothers is maintaining an adequate milk supply or dealing with an oversupply. While some women may struggle with producing enough milk, others may find themselves overwhelmed by excessive milk production, leading to engorgement and other discomforts.

Solution:

i. Establish a breastfeeding routine: Feed your baby frequently, following their hunger cues. Regular and frequent breastfeeding sessions help stimulate milk production and maintain an adequate supply.

ii. Ensure proper breastfeeding technique: Make sure your baby is effectively removing milk from the breasts by using proper latching and positioning techniques. This encourages milk production and prevents engorgement.

iii. Seek guidance from a lactation consultant: If you are experiencing low milk supply or oversupply issues, consulting with a lactation consultant can provide personalized guidance and support to address the problem.

Mastitis and Plugged Ducts:

Mastitis, which is the inflammation of breast tissue, and plugged ducts are common breastfeeding challenges that can cause pain, swelling, and flu-like symptoms. These conditions require prompt attention to prevent complications and maintain breastfeeding.

Solution:

i. Nurse frequently and effectively: Continuing to breastfeed or pump regularly helps keep the milk flowing and prevents clogged ducts. Ensure proper latching and feeding positions to ensure optimal milk drainage.

ii. Apply warm compresses: Applying warm compresses to the affected breast can help alleviate pain and promote milk flow. Gently massaging the area toward the nipple during feeding or pumping can also aid in relieving plugged ducts.

iii. Seek medical attention: If you suspect mastitis or have persistent plugged ducts, it is essential to consult a healthcare professional. They may prescribe antibiotics or recommend other interventions to resolve the issue.

B. Tips and Strategies for Overcoming Challenges

Proper Latching Techniques:

Mastering proper latching techniques is crucial for successful breastfeeding. It ensures effective milk transfer and reduces the risk of nipple soreness and other complications.

Solution:

i. Seek guidance from a lactation consultant: A lactation consultant can provide hands-on support and demonstrate proper latching techniques tailored to you and your baby's unique needs.

ii. Experiment with different positions: Explore different breastfeeding positions, such as the cradle hold, football hold, or side-lying position, to find what works best for you and your baby.

CHAPTER 3

Nutrition and Hydration for Breastfeeding Mothers

A. Dietary Considerations for Optimal Breastfeeding

Breastfeeding is an energy-demanding process that requires mothers to pay careful attention to their nutritional intake. Providing adequate calories and essential nutrients ensures the production of high-quality breast milk and supports the mother's overall health. Here are some key dietary considerations for optimal breastfeeding:

Adequate Calorie Intake:

During breastfeeding, a mother's calorie requirements increase to meet the energy demands of milk production. It is important to consume enough calories to maintain energy levels and support milk production.

On average, an additional 450-500 calories per day are recommended for breastfeeding mothers. However, individual calorie needs may vary based on factors such as body weight, activity level, and metabolism.

Balanced Diet with Essential Nutrients:

A well-balanced diet is crucial for breastfeeding mothers to ensure they receive all the necessary nutrients for their health and to pass on to their infants through breast milk. Include a variety of foods from the following groups:

Fruits and vegetables: These provide essential vitamins, minerals, and antioxidants.

Whole grains: Opt for whole grain bread, rice, pasta, and cereals to obtain fiber and B vitamins.

Lean proteins: Include lean meats, poultry, fish, legumes, and tofu for protein, iron, and zinc.

Healthy fats: Incorporate sources such as avocados, nuts, seeds, and olive oil for omega-3 fatty acids.

Dairy or alternatives: Choose low-fat dairy products or fortified plant-based milk for calcium and vitamin D.

Foods to Avoid or Limit:

Certain foods and substances can potentially affect the quality of breast milk or cause discomfort in infants. It is advisable for breastfeeding mothers to limit or avoid the following:

Caffeine: While moderate caffeine intake is generally considered safe, excessive consumption can make infants irritable or disrupt their sleep patterns. Limit your caffeine intake by monitoring your coffee, tea, soda, and chocolate consumption.

Alcohol: Alcohol can pass into breast milk and may negatively impact infant development. It is best to avoid alcohol or limit its consumption, ensuring it is fully metabolized before breastfeeding.

Strongly flavored or spicy foods: Some infants may be sensitive to strongly flavored or spicy foods, which can cause digestive issues or fussiness. Monitor your baby's reaction to such foods and adjust your diet accordingly.

B. Importance of Hydration for Milk Production

Staying adequately hydrated is essential for breastfeeding mothers as it supports milk production, prevents dehydration, and maintains overall health. Here's what you need to know about hydration:

Recommended Fluid Intake:

Aim to drink enough fluids throughout the day to quench your thirst and maintain hydration. While there is no specific formula for calculating fluid intake, a general guideline is to consume at least 8 to 10 cups (64-80 ounces) of fluids daily. Water is an excellent choice, but you can also include other beverages like milk, herbal teas, and fruit-infused water.

Hydration Tips for Breastfeeding Mothers:

Drink water before and after breastfeeding sessions to quench your thirst.

Keep a water bottle within reach during breastfeeding sessions and throughout the day as a reminder to stay hydrated.

Consume fluids with each meal and snack to ensure regular hydration.

If you find plain water boring, try infusing it with slices of citrus fruits or fresh herbs for a refreshing taste.

Limit the intake of sugary or caffeinated beverages, as they can have diuretic effects and may disrupt hydration levels.

Pay attention to your body's signals of thirst and drink whenever you feel thirsty.

Remember, every breastfeeding mother is unique.

CHAPTER 4

Exercise, the benefits and Physical Activity

A. Benefits of Exercise for Breastfeeding Mothers

Regular exercise and physical activity offer numerous benefits for breastfeeding mothers. Engaging in a well-planned exercise routine can positively impact both physical and mental well-being. Here are some key advantages of exercise for breastfeeding mothers:

Increased energy levels: Regular exercise can boost energy levels and combat fatigue, which is often experienced by new mothers. It helps improve overall stamina and promotes a sense of vitality, enabling mothers to better cope with the demands of breastfeeding and daily tasks.

Enhanced mood and mental well-being: Exercise stimulates the release of endorphins, also known as "feel-good" hormones, which can help alleviate symptoms of postpartum blues or depression. It promotes a positive mental state, reduces stress, and contributes to overall emotional well-being.

Weight management: Exercise plays a crucial role in weight management by aiding in the burning of calories and increasing metabolism. It can help breastfeeding mothers shed excess pregnancy weight while preserving lean muscle mass. However, it is essential to approach weight loss gradually and healthily, ensuring an adequate supply of nutrients for both mother and baby.

Improved cardiovascular health: Regular aerobic exercise, such as brisk walking, jogging, or swimming, helps strengthen the heart and improve cardiovascular fitness. This can have long-term benefits for breastfeeding mothers, reducing the risk of cardiovascular diseases and enhancing overall health and longevity.

Stress reduction: Exercise acts as a natural stress reliever and provides an opportunity for mothers to take time for themselves. Engaging in physical activity promotes relaxation, reduces anxiety, and allows for mental rejuvenation, ultimately leading to a better overall sense of well-being.

B. Safe Exercise Practices during Breastfeeding

While exercise is generally safe and beneficial for breastfeeding mothers, there are some important considerations to ensure both the mother's and baby's well-being.

Follow these safe exercise practices:

Consult with a healthcare professional: Before beginning any exercise program, consult with your healthcare provider or a certified fitness professional experienced in postpartum exercise. They can evaluate your situation, provide tailored advice, and address any specific concerns.

Start gradually and progress slowly: Begin with low-impact activities, such as walking or gentle stretching, and gradually increase the intensity and duration of your workouts over time. This allows your body to adapt and reduces the risk of injury or excessive strain.

Wear supportive clothing: Invest in a well-fitted, supportive sports bra to minimize discomfort and provide adequate breast support during exercise. Additionally, choose comfortable, breathable clothing that allows for freedom of movement.

Stay hydrated: It is essential to maintain proper hydration during exercise, especially while breastfeeding. Drink water before, during, and after your workout to replace fluids lost through sweat.

Listen to your body: Pay attention to how your body feels during and after exercise. If you experience pain, excessive fatigue, or any discomfort, it may be a sign to modify your routine or reduce the intensity. Always prioritize your comfort and well-being.

Consider breastfeeding or pumping before exercise: Breastfeed or pump milk before exercising to minimize breast discomfort, such as engorgement. This can also provide a more comfortable workout experience.

Monitor your baby's cues: Some babies may become fussy or refuse to breastfeed immediately after a mother's intense exercise session due to the taste of lactic acid in the milk. If this occurs, you can try breastfeeding before exercising or waiting for a while after your workout before offering milk.

Remember, every woman's postpartum recovery and breastfeeding journey is unique. Be mindful of your body's signals and adjust your exercise routine accordingly. By adopting safe exercise practices and gradually increasing your physical activity, you can enjoy the benefits of exercise while providing optimal care for yourself and your.

CHAPTER 5

Medication and Breastfeeding

A. Understanding the Safety of Medications during Breastfeeding

Breastfeeding mothers often have concerns about the safety of medications they may need to take while nursing their infants. This chapter aims to provide a comprehensive understanding of the safety considerations associated with medication use during breastfeeding.

Overview of Medication Transfer into Breast Milk

One of the primary concerns for breastfeeding mothers is whether medications can pass into breast milk and potentially affect the infant. While many medications can be detected in breast milk, the amount transferred is usually low and may not pose significant risks to the baby.

However, it is essential to assess each medication individually to determine its potential effects.

The transfer of medications into breast milk depends on several factors, such as the medication's chemical properties, maternal metabolism, and the infant's age and health. Additionally, the timing of medication administration relative to breastfeeding can impact the concentration of drugs in breast milk.

Factors Influencing Drug Safety:

Several factors influence the safety of medications during breastfeeding:

i. Medication Properties: Certain medications are known to pass more readily into breast milk, while others have limited transfer. Factors such as molecular size, lipid solubility, and protein binding can affect the amount of medication present in breast milk.

ii. Infant Age and Health: Newborns and premature infants may have reduced drug metabolism and elimination capabilities, making them more susceptible to potential medication effects. The health of the infant, including any existing medical conditions, should also be considered.

iii. Maternal Metabolism: The way medications are metabolized and eliminated from the mother's body can impact their presence in breast milk. Understanding how the body processes specific drugs can help determine their safety during breastfeeding.

B. Commonly Used Medications and Their Impact on Breastfeeding

Pain Relievers, Antibiotics, and Cold Medicines

Many over-the-counter pain relievers, antibiotics, and cold medicines are considered safe to use while breastfeeding. However, it is crucial to consult with a healthcare provider before taking any medication. Nonsteroidal anti-inflammatory drugs (NSAIDs) like ibuprofen and acetaminophen are generally considered safe choices for managing pain or fever during breastfeeding.

When it comes to antibiotics, certain types, such as penicillins, cephalosporins, and erythromycin, are commonly prescribed to breastfeeding mothers due to their low risk of causing harm to the infant.

While most cold medicines are considered safe, some ingredients, such as decongestants or antihistamines, may have mild effects on the infant, including drowsiness or a decrease in milk supply. It is important to carefully read labels and use medications as directed.

Antidepressants and Antianxiety Medications

Breastfeeding mothers who require treatment for depression or anxiety have several options available. Selective serotonin reuptake inhibitors (SSRIs), such as sertraline and escitalopram, are commonly prescribed due to their relatively low levels in breast milk and minimal impact on infants.

While SSRIs are generally considered safe, it is essential to monitor the baby for any unusual symptoms. Healthcare providers may also consider alternative medications or adjunct therapies if necessary.

Chronic Disease Management Medications

Mothers with chronic diseases like hypertension, asthma, or diabetes may need to continue taking medications during breastfeeding. Most medications used for chronic disease management have been studied extensively, and the risks to the infant are often outweighed by the benefits of breastfeeding.

Consulting with healthcare providers is crucial for individualized advice on medication choices and any necessary adjustments to ensure the safety of both mother and baby.

CHAPTER 6

Weaning from Breastfeeding

A. Signs of Readiness for Weaning

Weaning is a significant milestone in a baby's life and can be an emotional journey for both mother and child. Recognizing the signs of readiness for weaning is crucial in ensuring a smooth transition. While every child is unique, here are some common indicators that your baby may be ready to start the weaning process:

Age and Development: Most experts recommend waiting until your baby is at least six months old before initiating weaning. By this age, babies have typically developed the necessary skills to eat solid foods and rely less on breast milk for their nutritional needs.

Interest in Solid Foods: If your baby shows curiosity about what you're eating, tries to grab food from your plate, or mimics chewing motions, it may be a sign that they are ready to explore new tastes and textures.

Decreased Nursing Frequency: If your baby naturally starts spacing out their nursing sessions or seems less interested in breastfeeding, it may indicate that they are ready for a gradual reduction in breast milk intake.

Acceptance of Bottles or Cups: If your baby has successfully transitioned to drinking from a bottle or sippy cup, it shows that can adapt to alternative feeding methods, which is an essential step towards weaning.

Independent Eating Skills: As your baby develops better motor skills and can self-feed with a spoon or their fingers, it becomes easier to introduce solid foods and gradually reduce breast milk intake.

B. Different Weaning Methods and Approaches

There are various weaning methods and approaches, and choosing the right one depends on your baby's needs and circumstances. Here are some commonly used approaches:

Gradual Weaning: This method involves gradually replacing breastfeeding sessions with solid foods or formula. Start by substituting one breastfeeding session per day with a bottle or cup feeding. Over time, continue to replace additional sessions until your baby is fully weaned.

Child-Led Weaning: With this approach, you allow your baby to self-wean at their own pace. Your role is to provide nutritious foods and respond to their cues. Child-led weaning is typically a gentle and gradual process that respects the baby's readiness to let go of breastfeeding.

Mother-Led Weaning: In this method, the mother takes the lead in initiating and guiding the weaning process. It involves gradually reducing breastfeeding sessions and replacing them with other sources of nutrition. This approach can be helpful when there are time constraints or health considerations.

Combination Weaning: Some mothers choose to combine breastfeeding with bottle or cup feeding to gradually transition their baby to alternative sources of nutrition. This method allows for flexibility and can be tailored to suit individual needs.

C. Managing Emotional Aspects of Weaning for Both Mother and Baby

Weaning is not just a physical transition but an emotional one as well, both for the mother and the baby. Here are some strategies to manage the emotional aspects of weaning:

Communication and Preparation:

Talk to your baby about the upcoming changes and explain that breastfeeding will be gradually reduced. Maintain a nurturing and loving environment, assuring your baby that they will still receive ample love and care during the weaning process.

Comfort and Distraction: Offer comfort and distractions when your baby seeks breastfeeding for emotional support. Engage in activities together, such as playing, reading, or cuddling, to redirect their attention.

Support System: Seek support from your partner, family, or friends during this emotional journey. Discuss your feelings with someone who understands and can provide encouragement and reassurance.

Weaning can be an emotional time for mothers as well.

CHAPTER 7

Self-Care and Support for Breastfeeding Mothers

Congratulations, breastfeeding mother! By reaching this chapter, you have already embarked on an incredible journey of providing the best nutrition and bonding experience for your baby. However, it is crucial to remember that taking care of yourself is just as important as caring for your little one. In this chapter, we will explore the significance of self-care during breastfeeding and the importance of seeking and building a support network. By prioritizing your well-being and surrounding yourself with a supportive community, you can enhance your breastfeeding experience and promote your overall health.

A. Importance of Self-Care during Breastfeeding:

Physical Self-Care:

i. Adequate Rest: Breastfeeding can be demanding, and it is essential to prioritize rest and sleep. When possible, try to nap when your baby sleeps, delegate household chores, and ask for help from your partner or loved ones.

ii. Balanced Nutrition: Your body requires additional nutrients during breastfeeding. Focus on consuming a well-balanced diet rich in fruits, vegetables, whole grains, lean proteins, and healthy fats. Stay hydrated by drinking plenty of water throughout the day.

iii. Gentle Exercise: Engaging in light exercise can boost your energy levels and promote overall well-being. Consult with your healthcare provider about suitable postpartum exercises that are safe for you and your baby, such as gentle walks or yoga.

iv. Personal Hygiene: Taking care of your physical appearance, such as showering regularly, can boost your mood and self-confidence.

Emotional Self-Care:

i. Recognize and Express Your Feelings: Breastfeeding can bring a range of emotions, from joy and contentment to frustration and exhaustion. Allow yourself to acknowledge and express these feelings openly. Talk to your partner, friends, or a healthcare professional if you need emotional support.

ii. Engage in Relaxation Techniques: Incorporate relaxation techniques into your daily routine, such as deep breathing exercises, meditation, or listening to calming music. These practices can help reduce stress and anxiety.

iii. Pursue Hobbies and Interests: Carve out time for activities that bring you joy and fulfillment. Engaging in hobbies or pursuing personal interests can provide a sense of accomplishment and help maintain your identity outside of motherhood.

B. Seeking and Building a Support Network:

Partner Support:

i. Communicate Openly: Share your breastfeeding goals and challenges with your partner. Mutual understanding and support can strengthen your bond and make the breastfeeding journey more enjoyable.

ii. Encourage Participation: Involve your partner in the breastfeeding process. They can assist with tasks like burping the baby, diaper changes, or offering support during nighttime feedings.

Family and Friends:

i. Educate Your Loved Ones: Inform your family and friends about the importance of breastfeeding and the challenges you may face. Encourage them to learn and understand the benefits, so they can offer appropriate support and encouragement.

ii. Seek Assistance: Don't hesitate to ask for help when needed. Loved ones can provide practical support, such as preparing meals, helping with household chores, or babysitting, allowing you to have some much-needed rest.

Join Support Groups:

i. Local Breastfeeding Support Groups: Look for local breastfeeding support groups where you can connect with other breastfeeding mothers. These groups provide a safe space to share experiences, seek advice, and receive emotional support from individuals who understand the challenges and joys of breastfeeding.

ii. Online Communities: Explore online forums and communities dedicated to breastfeeding. These virtual spaces offer a vast network of experienced mothers who can provide guidance, answer questions, and offer words of encouragement.

Conclusion:

As a breastfeeding mother, it is crucial to prioritize self-care and build a robust support network. By taking care of your physical and emotional well-being.

SUMMARY

Embracing Breastfeeding for Women's Health: A Pathway to Well-being

Throughout this book, we have explored the numerous benefits of breastfeeding for both the baby and the mother. As we summarize this journey, it's essential to recap the remarkable advantages that breastfeeding offers to women's health.

Breastfeeding is a powerful ally in promoting maternal well-being. It not only provides essential nutrients to the newborn but also supports the mother's physical and emotional health. Studies have shown that breastfeeding can reduce the risk of certain health conditions for women, including:

Reduced risk of breast cancer: Breastfeeding has been linked to a decreased risk of developing breast cancer. The longer a woman breastfeeds, the more significant the risk reduction. By nourishing their infants through breastfeeding, mothers are taking an active step towards safeguarding their health.

Lowered risk of ovarian cancer: Breastfeeding has also been associated with a reduced risk of ovarian cancer. The hormonal changes that occur during breastfeeding contribute to this protective effect. By choosing to breastfeed, mothers provide themselves a potential shield against this potentially life-threatening disease.

Postpartum recovery: Breastfeeding stimulates the release of oxytocin, which helps the uterus contract and return to its pre-pregnancy size. This natural process assists in the healing and recovery of the mother's body after childbirth, reducing the risk of postpartum complications.

Weight management: Breastfeeding burns extra calories, aiding mothers in their efforts to lose pregnancy weight. It provides a gentle, sustainable approach to weight management, promoting a healthy body composition while also reducing the risk of obesity-related health issues in the long term.

Improved mental health: The act of breastfeeding fosters a profound emotional bond between mother and child, which can have a positive impact on the mother's mental well-being. Breastfeeding releases hormones like oxytocin and prolactin, promoting relaxation, stress reduction, and a sense of fulfillment and happiness.

Encouragement for Mothers to Embrace Breastfeeding for Their Well-being

Mothers, as you have journeyed through the pages of this book, you have gained valuable insight into the immense benefits that breastfeeding holds for your health. I want to take this moment to encourage and empower you to embrace breastfeeding for your well-being.

Remember that your health matters, and by choosing to breastfeed, you are making a conscious decision to prioritize it. Breastfeeding is not only an act of nourishment but an act of self-care. It is a gift you give to yourself, allowing your body to heal, thrive, and flourish.

Embrace the beauty of the breastfeeding journey. It may have its challenges, but remember that you are not alone. Seek support from your partner, family, friends, and healthcare professionals who can provide guidance and assistance along the way. Surround yourself with a nurturing network that celebrates and supports your decision to breastfeed.

Find solace in the knowledge that you are creating a strong foundation for your health, both in the present and for the future. Breastfeeding is a transformative experience that not only benefits you but also creates a lasting bond with your child. It is an investment in their health and well-being, and it sets the stage for a brighter and healthier future for both of you.

Finally;

I encourage you to continue seeking knowledge and support on this topic. There are numerous resources available that can provide you with additional information, guidance, and a sense of community:

Reach out to certified lactation consultants who specialize in breastfeeding support. They can provide personalized guidance, and address any concerns or challenges you may face.